Controlling Child Obesity

Keeping Your Children Healthy

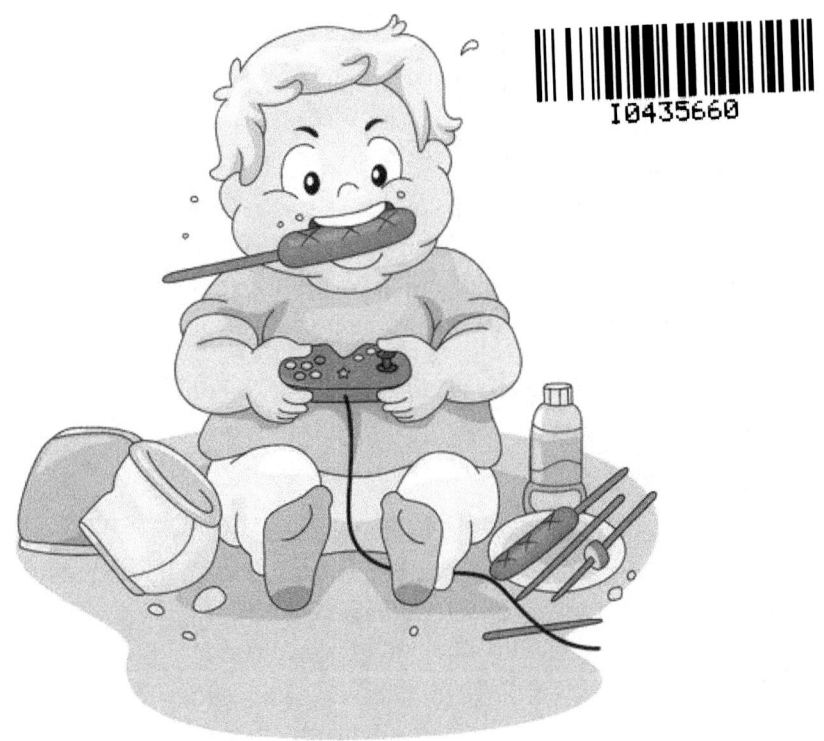

Natural Health Series

Dueep J. Singh

Mendon Cottage Books

JD-Biz Publishing

Disclaimer

The information is this book is provided for informational purposes only. It is not intended to be used and medical advice or a substitute for proper medical treatment by a qualified health care provider. The information is believed to be accurate as presented based on research by the author.

The contents have not been evaluated by the U.S. Food and Drug Administration or any other Government or Health Organization and the contents in this book are not to be used to treat cure or prevent disease.

The author or publisher is not responsible for the use or safety of any diet, procedure or treatment mentioned in this book. The author or publisher is not responsible for errors or omissions that may exist.

Warning

The Book is for informational purposes only and before taking on any diet, treatment or medical procedure, it is recommended to consult with your primary health care provider.

Check out some of the other Healthy Gardening Series books at Amazon.com

Gardening Series on Amazon

Check out some of the other Health Learning Series books at Amazon.com

Health Learning Series on Amazon

Table of Contents

Introduction

Did you know that in the last 30 years, the childhood obesity cases in children have more than doubled and more than quadrupled, in teenagers and adolescents, in the USA alone?

7% of children were considered to be obese in 1980. In 2012, that percentage had increased to 18%. In the same manner, teenage obesity had increased from 5% to 21% in that particular time period.

What is the difference between obesity and overweight? Overweight means that our body has extra body weight, due to water, bone, fat, muscle, or any of these combined factors for a particular and given height. On the other hand, obesity is concerned with just extra body fat.

Millennium ago, the idea of children being obese was a rather rare phenomenon. They may have been overweight, because of lack of physical exercise and eating lots of food indiscriminately. But they were not obese, because they were not genetically conditioned to be so. Also, sedentary lifestyles at that time was not encouraged in children because, since childhood, they were trained to do hard physical labor, which they would continue for the rest of their lives.

In many parts of the world, there are still societies which equate being fat and well-rounded with being prosperous. That is the reason why even now, mothers still stuff up their children, with lots and lots of food, so that people do not blame them for "starving their children" because they are so thin.

How did this attitude of society come into being? We have to go back millenniums ago, when man was still struggling to survive. That is when it was not so easy for him to get enough of food to feed his large family. This is the reason why plenty of his children stayed hungry unless they could forage for themselves.

It was only in a comparatively prosperous family, that they could get enough of food to eat, in order to get "fat." That is when fat became synonymous with prosperity. Kings and emperors were never shown to be lean, slim and thin, unless they were warriors and were in battle worthy conditions, in wall paintings or rock carvings. They had this bit of a paunch.

This was to show that they had enough of food to eat and to eat heartily, so that they could get fat.

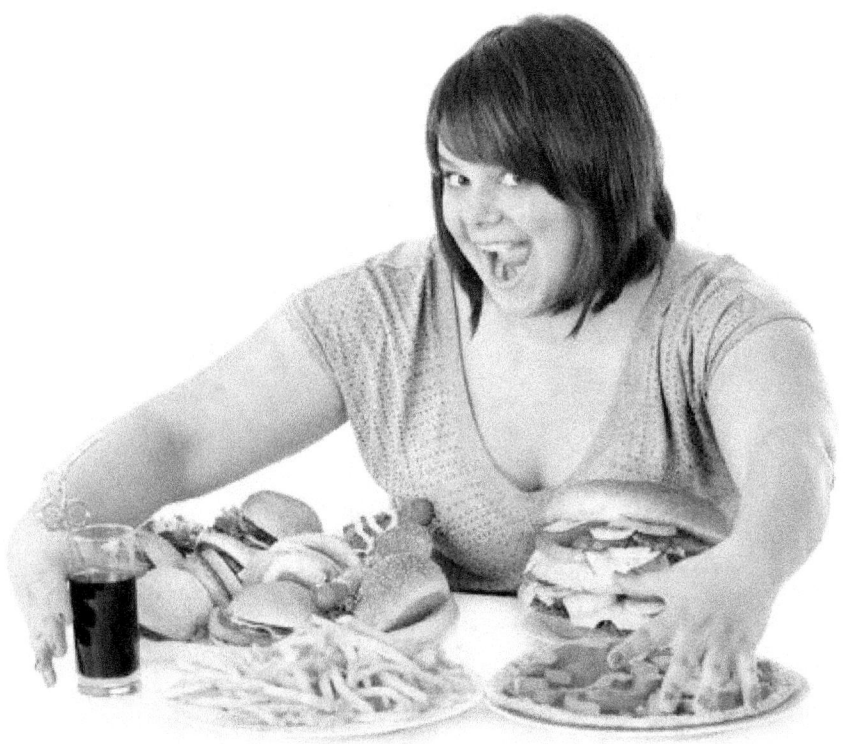

Reasons for obesity

Caloric imbalance is the reason why people suffer from obesity and overweight. This means that you are expending too few calories in the form of "burning off calories" in proportion to the amounts of calories eaten in your diet. Also, environmental, behavioral, genetic and dietary factors are going to influence your health, possibly causing obesity and overweight problems.

Side effects of Childhood Obesity

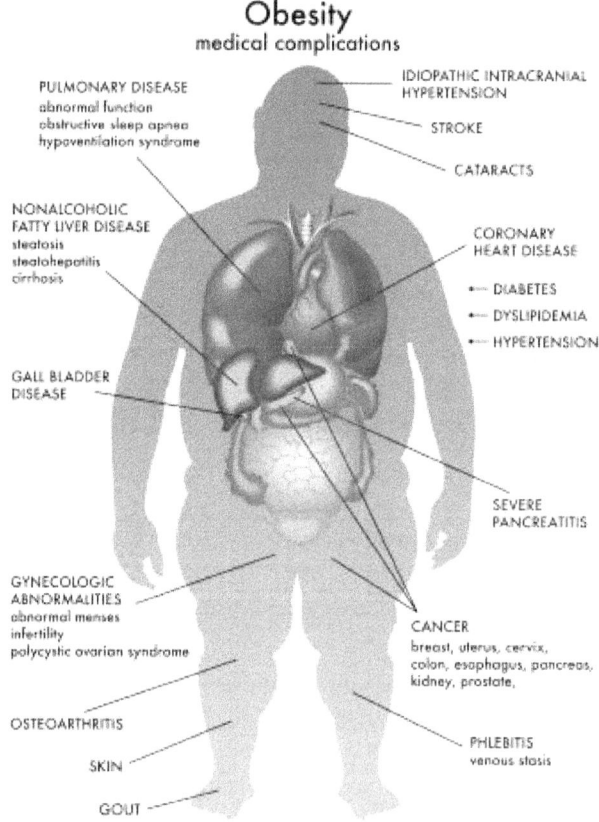

Obesity
medical complications

Childhood obesity is definitely going to have a long-term effect on your general health, especially when you reach adulthood. If bad eating habits have made you obese as a child, you are going to suffer from potential heart problems, and other weight related problems when you grow up. These also include high blood pressure, high cholesterol levels, possibility of diabetes, and joint problems.

Along with that, a child who is obese is going to suffer from an inferiority complex, as well as poor self-confidence and self-esteem. He is going to be targeted among his peers, with nicknames like "potato", "hippopotamus" or "fatty" depending on the imagination of his companions, and friends.

This is going to lead to psychological as well as social problems. This is because society considers being fat to be synonymous with being unattractive. It is only in Papua New Guinea, and other islands in the sun, where fat women are considered to be beautiful.

In olden times, in the East, fat women were considered to be the epitome of beauty and maharajas, Sheikhs and Sultans married sultanas with Juno-esque and goddess like proportions, because that was the idea of Earth mother goddess in those far-off days. But those body proportions were considered to be beautiful in adults and not in children.

Children were considered beautiful, when they were slim , lithe and trim in shape, instead of being little butter balls. And that is why obesity was not encouraged in children and youth, down the ages.

However, thanks to bad eating habits, and changes in lifestyle, those childhood days, where children spend their childhood, enjoying plenty of outdoor activities, especially climbing up trees, fishing in ponds and pools, and getting into scrapes has unfortunately now become restricted to nostalgic stories

The average modern child is going to be found dining off chips and burgers, and sitting hunched in front of a computer or in front of the TV, watching cartoons. His posture is going to be slumped, as he watches anorexic movie stars, – suffering from eating disorders, due to excessive dieting – bouncing all around the floor, or space monsters coming down to attack planet Earth.

This change in habits has thus led to changes in the health of children during the past 30 years or so. There is a word generation, now, which is predominantly an obese one, because of bad eating habits. Poor food choices, sedentary lifestyles, and not enough knowledge about nutritional eating has led to either anorexia or obesity in children.

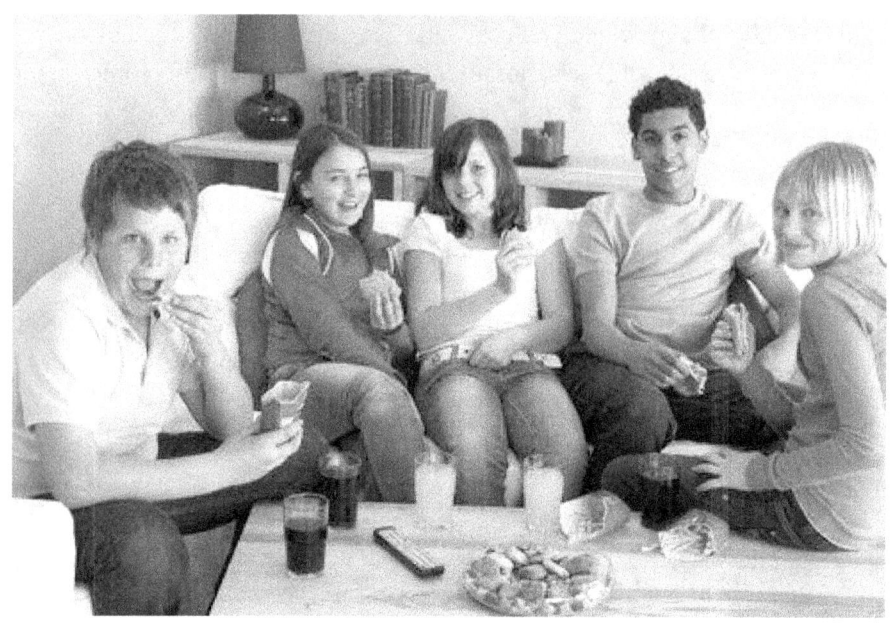

Sedentary lifestyles and bad eating habits means future weight problems.

Childhood obesity has been directly linked to cardiovascular diseases because the fatty deposits that lead to such diseases start accumulating right in childhood itself.

Overprotective parents in this modern day and age, do not allow their children to cycle or walk to school. One is the acceptable reason of child safety. The other is that they do not bother about telling their children about how necessary physical exercises are for their well-being.

Children would rather travel in cars or in buses instead of walking or cycling.

In the last 10 years, the number of overweight children under the age of four have increase anywhere from one sixth to one quarter in many parts of the world, while obesity has doubled to nearly 1 in 10, when once it was 1 in 50 or even 75.

That is because the number of calories being consumed by an average child has increased by more than 200, while those calories are definitely not being burnt off.

So once you know all about the relationship between calorie intake and obesity, you need to look at the source of calories eaten. The necessary nutrients needed to keep you healthy, which include vitamins and minerals should be added in your daily diet right now.

If foods are eaten, which are poor providers of these necessary ingredients, the overall energy and health level of a child is going to be affected. He is going to suffer from anemia, due to vitamin deficiency. He is also going to be lethargic and non-energetic.

Does Your Child Have a Genuine Weight Problem?

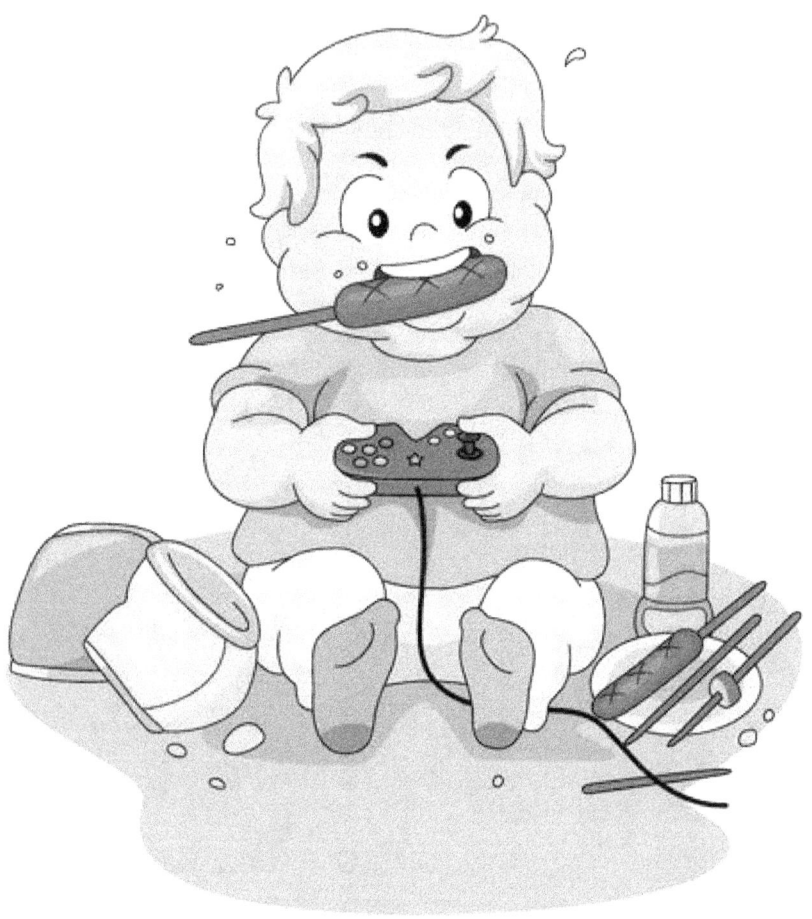

Believe it or not, I have come across parents, who definitely do not want to believe that their children have a genuine weight problem. According to them, their children are healthy, where I consider them to be overweight or even frankly obese. That is because these parents have been brought up conditioned with a mindset that a happy, healthy child is that one which is well padded out and roly-poly.

Whether they know it or not, these parents are doing their best to win the natural good health of their children, because of their ignorance or because of their stubbornness.

An adult body mass index calculator chart, available at your doctor is not going to work for children. So you need to measure it on a pediatric's guide chart. They are going to have the appropriate growth charts for children and for babies. You can look for them on the Internet, depending on the age of your child.

This is an excellent URL. A youth, older than 20 years will need an adult chart.

http://nccd.cdc.gov/dnpabmi/

How to prevent Obesity in Your Child

There was a time when parents spent enough of time, outdoors, indulging in pleasant activities like walking, camping, tennis, swimming, and other physical activities, along with their children. But nowadays, parents are so busy, that they have forgotten about taking part in such activities. If you cannot play with your child, every day, outdoors, you can at least spend some time in weekend sports, in a whole family group.

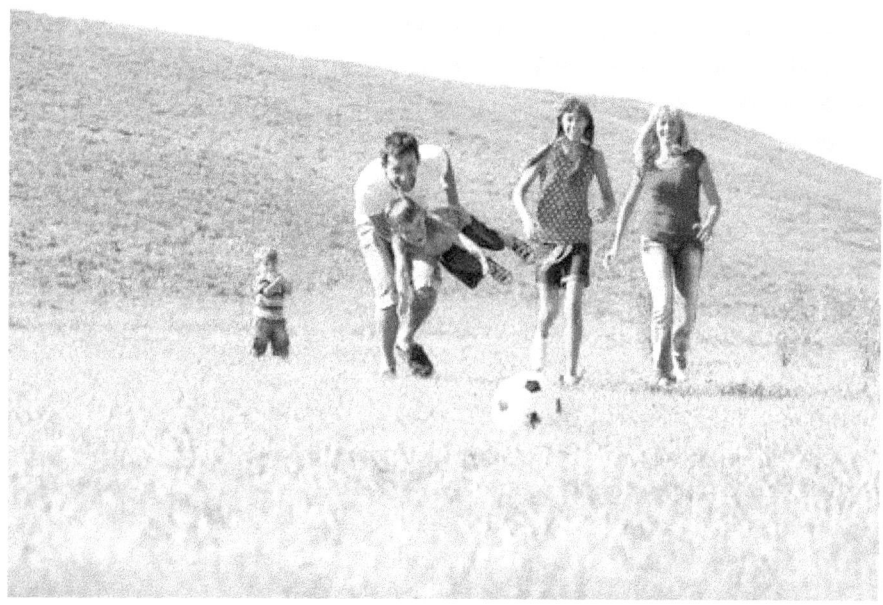

The family that plays together stays together...

Not only is this going to be quality time spent with your children, but this is part of social and family bonding. You can join clubs for physical activities which you are going to do together.

If children are not getting enough of opportunities to play games every day at school, they need to be encouraged to spend at least one hour outside in the fresh air and sun.

A child who knows and learns the value of sports since childhood is going to be a healthy active teenager and adult.

Cut back on all the sedentary activities like watching TV or playing video or computer games. This is where parents have to be strict. I know a number of parents, who are happy, that their children are sitting quietly in their rooms, playing games, instead of bothering them in noisy activity. This mindset is definitely not a proper one.

You may need to limit TV and computer games to 60 minutes on school days, and up to 90 minutes daily during holidays and weekends. A little bit of discipline, now means that you are not going to have children who come under the couch potato category.

If the parents are suffering from weight problems, there is a chance that the child is also going to be vulnerable to such a problem. That is because either this problem is genetically inherited, or it has been caused due to the bad eating habits of the parents.

Do not put children on slimming diets which are tailored for adults. Children have different nutritional requirements. They are in their growing since, that is why they need all the minerals, vitamins, proteins, carbohydrates, and other nutrients necessary to keep their bodies healthy. They are in their growing stage, and that is why any paucity of these nutrients is going to have a harmful long-term aftereffect in their bodies.

On the other hand, an adult can get away without having a couple of meals or meals in reduced quantities or meals which do not have some ingredients in the essential four food groups. You cannot afford to take this risk with children. They need plenty of nutritious food, at regular intervals.

That is why you need to teach your child all about healthy eating, right from the very beginning itself. At the same time, you need to start changing your own eating habits so that your children start accepting healthy meals as a part of their daily routine.

The breakfast cereals that you get in the market today are full of sugary items. Instead, you would want to change the breakfast menu to whole-wheat toast, homemade pancakes, boiled eggs, and even porridge.

Children should be given fresh juice at breakfast

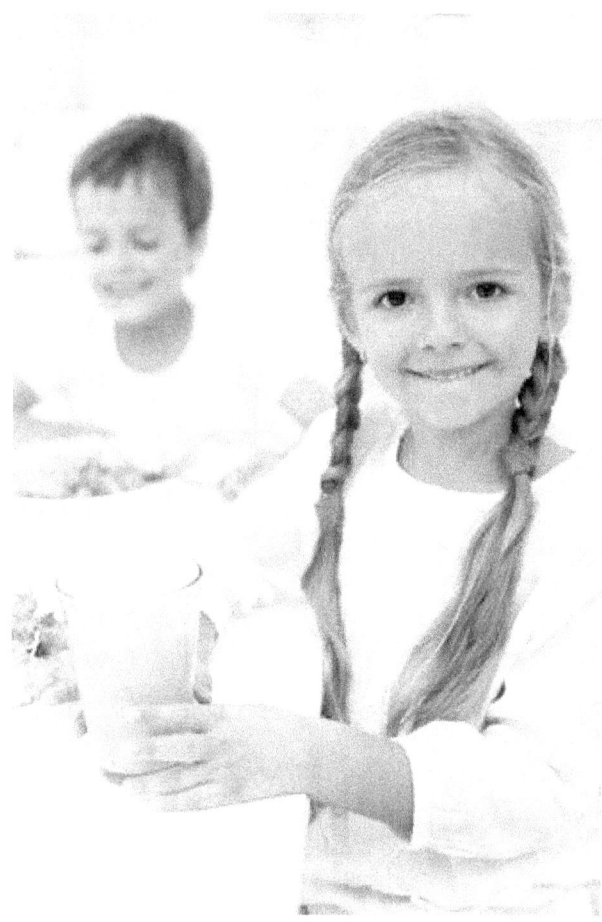

For snacks, to be eaten at school, you can pack in mini sandwiches with plenty of greens, cheese, etc. Accompanying these sandwiches, you can add cauliflower flowers, green beans, raw carrots sticks and baby tomatoes.Put all of them in a hamburger. Your kids are going to eat them, because according to them, hamburgers come under the category of junk food and anything in a hamburger is acceptable! A child psychologist told me this! Spice up the hamburger with herbs, and garlic salt.

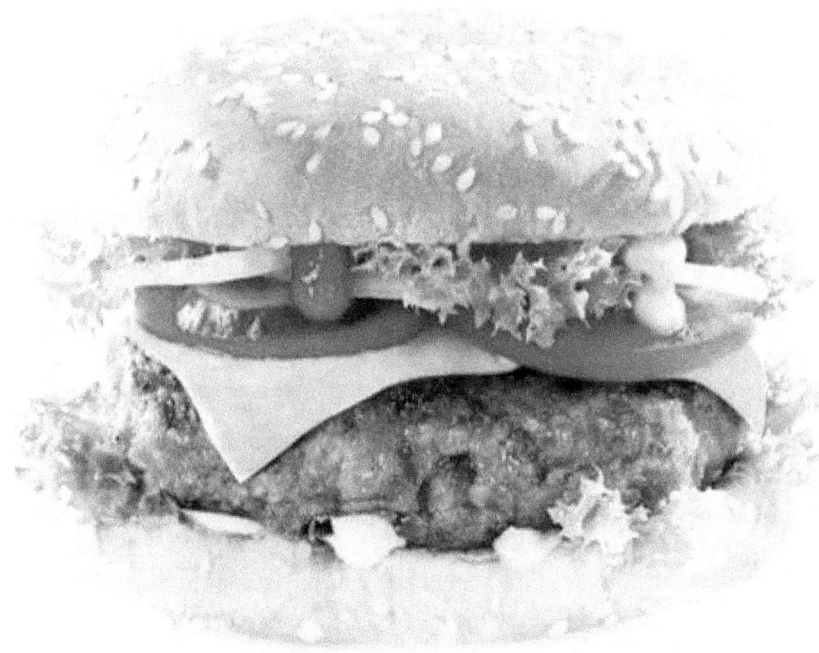

Do not stop your children from having chips and junk food at school. Not only is this impractical, but it is impossible. You may, however, teach them the value of smaller helpings.

Grilled chicken kebabs and pizzas made at home with all the vegetables given above are going to be eaten by your children, if they have a sprinkling of cheese on them. Encourage your children to help you cook these meals, because they are going to like eating them. Get them to put their own choice of ingredients on their individual pizzas.

Apart from eating fruit raw, these fruit can also be given to them, in pies and custards as well as other dessert preparations, which include fruit.

If you concentrate on healthy eating at home, and remember to keep your fridge and kitchen stocked with healthy food items, they are not going to be stuffing themselves on potato chips, crisps, and sweets. Processed foods are also definitely not healthy, so cut out the processed cheeses and processed meats from your diet list.

Cannot do without meat? Get it straight from the butchers and freshly cut. Do not go in for marketed and packaged brands, because they are going to have plenty of artificial preservatives.

Make some ground rules for eating in your family now. No proper time structure for mealtimes means that children are either going to skip meals, or they are going to have meals at awkward times. Eat regularly, along with your children. If you cannot manage to eat your meals together at the kitchen table, eat them someplace else, where you can see your children eating a healthy meal.

No snacking – in the 21st century, healthy food items are being replaced by low nutrient easy to eat foods. These include soft drinks, colas, squashes and concentrated juice drinks. Teach your children the harm these drinks are going to do to their internal systems, as well as to their teeth. This is going to stop them from drinking these potentially dangerous drinks.

Do not keep these drinks at home. Instead, you may want to encourage them to drink water or fresh fruit juice. Children should under no circumstances be put on to coffee or tea. This is not only a foolish habit, but it is also going to ruin their health, because of the caffeine and tannin intake.

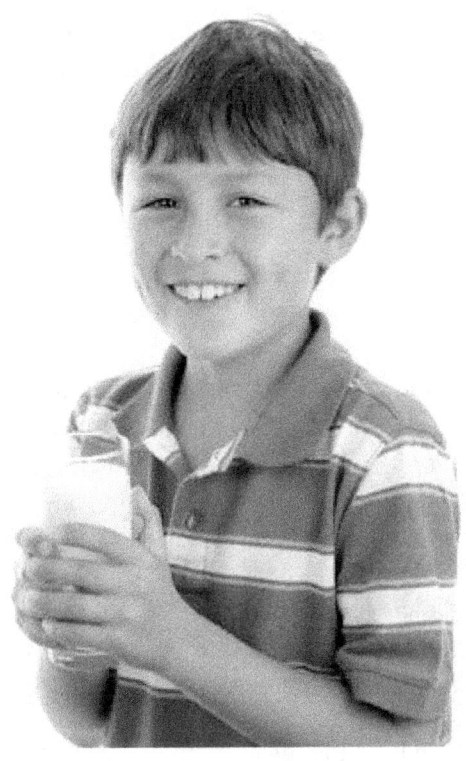

The best drink for a growing child is, of course, a glassful of milk, twice a day. You may want to add honey to it. Do not add chemical-based milk products, which are being branded by companies as delicious chocolate flavored malt milk products, healthy for your children. They are not healthy. That is because they have artificial preservatives in them.

Healthy Convenience Food Options

Even though I am not an advocate of convenience foods, it is possible that in most cases, parents make do with convenience foods to feed their children, because they just cannot manage to make fresh meals every day. That is the reason why you need to look at all the convenience food options, which are healthier and nutritious.

If you are serving burgers and sausages, you need to limit their servings, about two times a week. If your children are eating out at their school canteen, it is possible that sausages and burgers are going to be a part of the school menu. So to boost up the nutritional value of these meat products, add fruit and vegetables to the diet.

Did you know that more than USD800 million are being spent annually on ready-made pizzas, meat products, and sausages? Believe it or not, USD1.9 billion in the USA alone are being spent on ready to eat packed meals. All of these meals are high in fat and salt content, and low in nutrients.

Be very selective about what you intend to buy. Make intelligent substitutions by looking at the ingredient list. Many of these products are made up of fillers and fat. Look for meat items which have 85% more meat when compared to 65% meat, and the rest preservatives and fillers.

Potato chips – if you have to buy any, should be easy to bake or thickly cut. Look for potato chips, which can be grilled or baked in an oven , instead of being fried in hot grease.

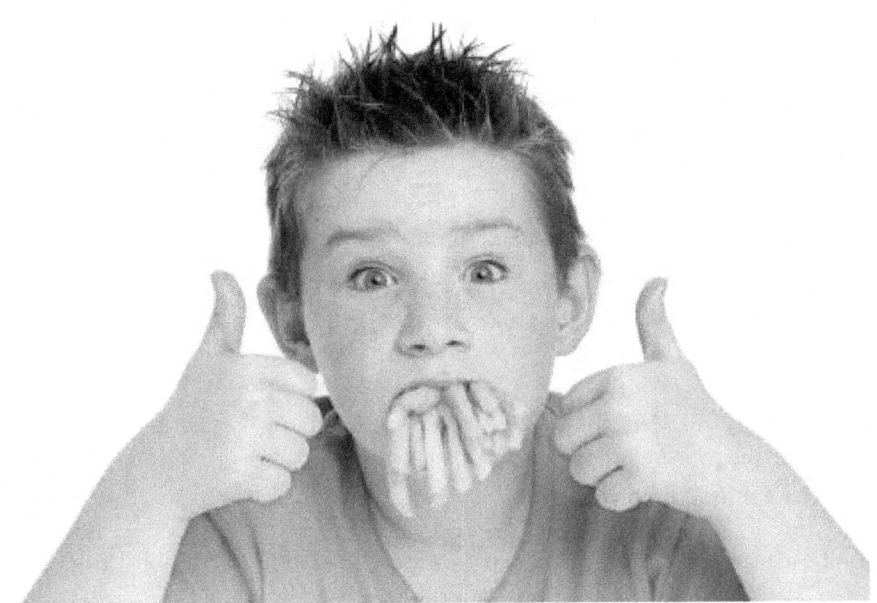

This occasional stuffing of his face is acceptable if these chips were baked or grilled.

Soups – world-famous soups like Campbell and Knorr may taste delicious, but they are very high in salt and preservative content. Homemade soup is always better, because you know exactly what you are putting in it. Serve this soup with whole meal rolls instead of refined white bread.

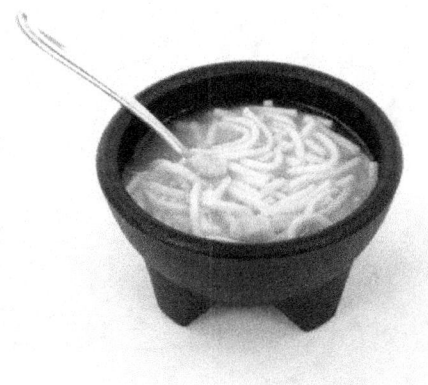

There is nothing like homemade soup, with noodles added to boost up the natural immunity system of your children, in a healthy manner. Chicken soup is best.

Meat products – if you really have to buy meat products, look for those products, which have 85% meat. Better still, buy hundred percent meat, fresh from your butchers. Mass-produced greasy sausages are getting to be very common today, so look for places where you can get really meaty and juicy sausages.

If you have a farm nearby, you are lucky, because they are not going to be putting in preservatives in their ham, bacon or other meat products. This may come to be a bit more expensive, but in the general scheme of things, this is a much more healthy option.

Fish and chips – this is one of the staple foods, in England. Parents going back home after a hard days' work just drop into the nearest take away, and order fish and chips. Fish and chips, five days a week for dinner is definitely not healthy. You may want to eat it, sometimes for a treat.

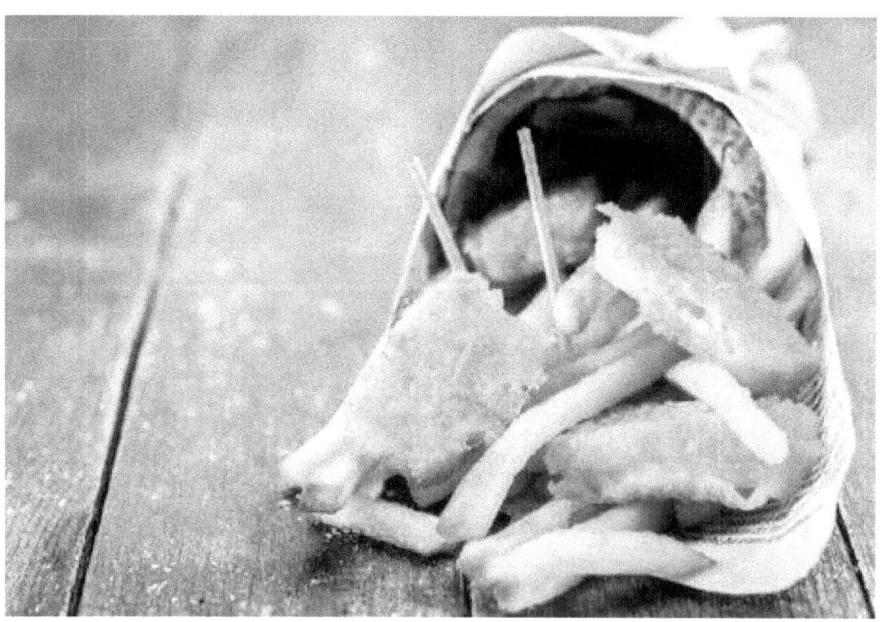

Pull off some of the greasy batter and add beans and peas for more nutrition. The overall fat content of fish and chips found in the supermarket is definitely going to be lesser than that fried in front of you in the friendly neighborhood fish and chips stall.

Beans – beans, especially when they are baked can be considered to be a healthy convenience food. Look for those bean products, which are low on salt and low on sugar. Serve them with whole grain toast.

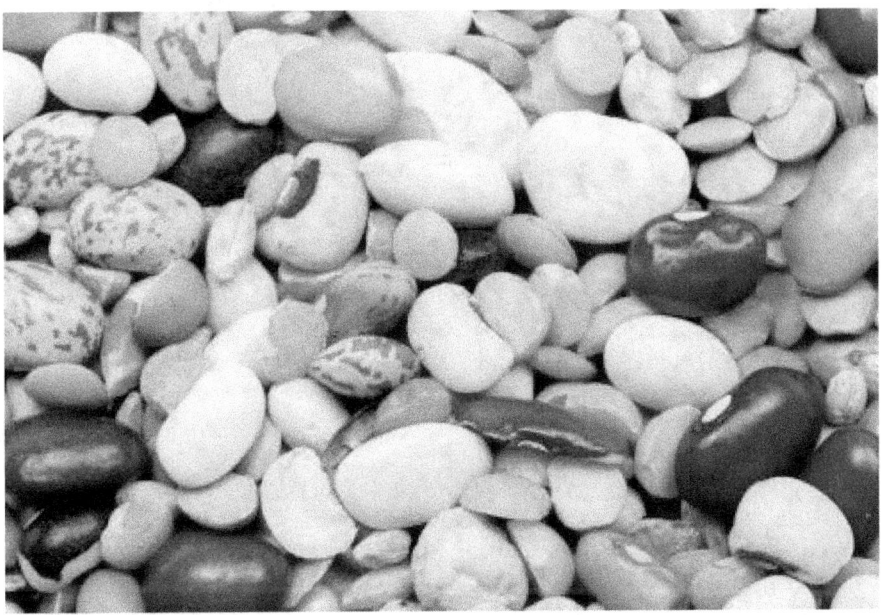

Pasta – many of us cannot do without pasta and macaroni. This is going to be a healthy option as long as it is not smothered in creamy sauce. Look for pasta with tomato-based sauces.

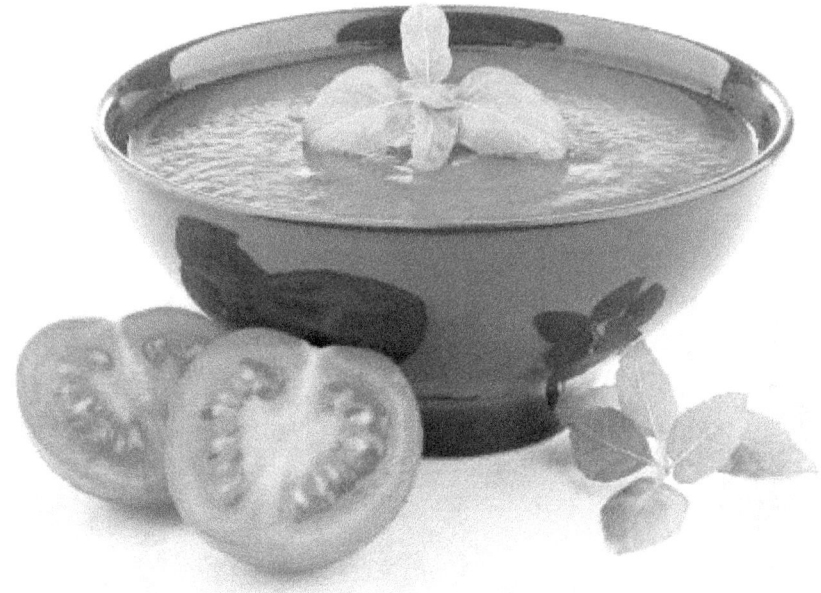

 Add some vegetables like broccoli, cauliflower, tomatoes and other raw vegetables to the wok and stirfry slowly with herbs, to make it more nutritional, before serving.

Cannot do without pizza? Add sliced tomatoes and cut up vegetables as extra layers on pizza. Look for thin crust pizzas because thick crust pizzas are going to have extra cheese in them.

Homemade Burger Patties

2 pounds of ground meat – pork or veal for choice – from the butchers.

Your favorite combination of herbs, including 2 teaspoons of sage, a teaspoon full of marjoram and thyme, three fourths of a teaspoon of cayenne pepper, 2 teaspoons full of salt, and half a teaspoon of pepper. Add any other herbs you like. I normally add two – three cloves of crushed garlic, one small onion, a sprig of parsley chopped up, and any other herb I have at hand, including mint

Mixing is normally done by putting all these ingredients in a bowl, and kneading and squeezing it the old-fashioned way, with your hands. Somehow the modern way of putting it in a blender and allowing to blend does not give the mixture that same unique blended taste which you get through hand mixing.

For a good flavored hamburger, you must know your herbs and whether they are fresh or not. Grow your own herbs, if possible, on your kitchen windowsill.

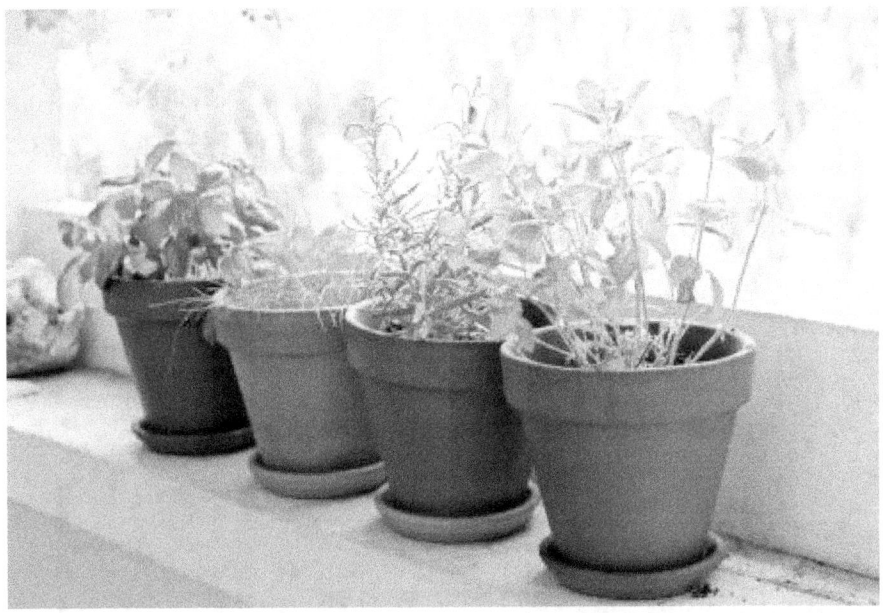

Shape the mixed mixture into patties, dust with flour, and grill on a hot griddle or on a skillet. Use the minimum of grease for frying, if you are frying them. Grilled meat is better, as long as you know that it has been cooked well.

If you are using the skillet and have just fried the burgers, you may want to swirl a little hot water around in the skillet, to gather up the crackling and fat. This tasty gravy is going to taste really nice, when eaten with bread or poured on those patties which you have not used to make up hamburgers.

You can also try making chicken burgers by chopping up chicken breast meat, and add an Apple. Chop 30 g of onions, and add 200 g of your preferred meat,cut into chunks. Blend on high speed until they are finely chopped. We do not want mushy breast meat. You can also make this with lean pork meat, and add apples and pears.

Add your favorite herbs. Form into patties, bake, fry or grill with a little bit of olive oil on medium heat, make sure that it is thoroughly cooked.

Serve on buns, with chopped greens, salad, sour cream, and Relish.

The patties which are extra, and uncooked can be frozen for use whenever you want.

Homemade chicken Nuggets

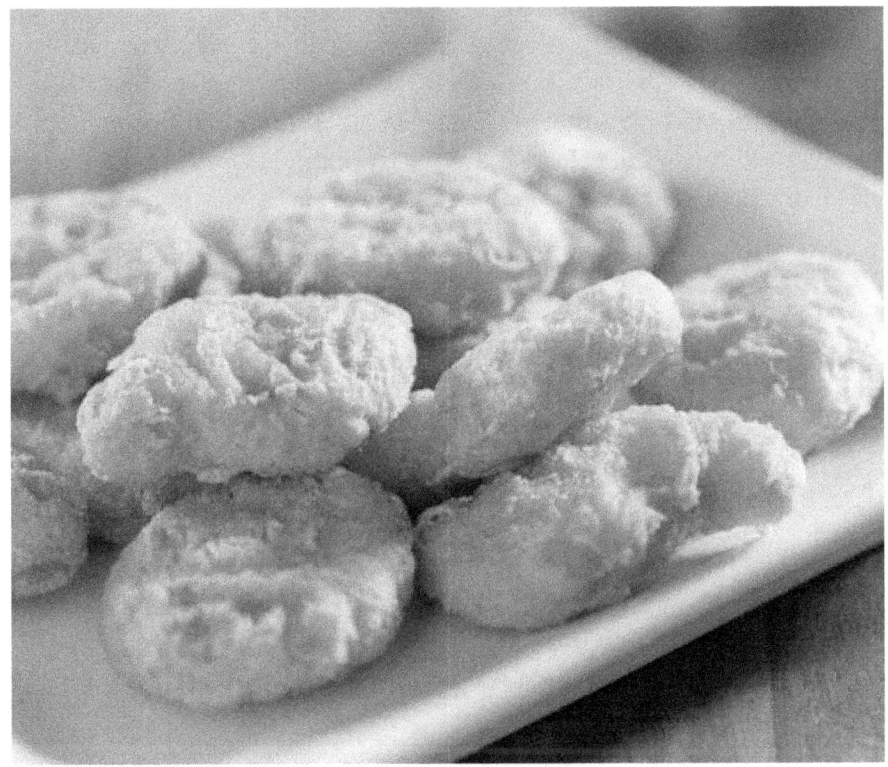

If your children really enjoy chicken nuggets, it is much better to make them at home, with bread crumbs made up of three slices of bread, put in a bowl and seasoned with your own favorite herbs and spices. Then beat two eggs in another small bowl. Cut three or four chicken breast fillets into long strips. Dunk the fillets one by one in the egg, and then into the breadcrumbs so that if they are properly coated on all sides.

Now, heat some oil in a frying pan. I normally use a wok because that is going to give me equally hot areas all over the surface of the utensil. Fry them for about 10 minutes until they are cooked thoroughly on all sides.

These can be par – cooked more gently until cooked through but not completely browned, and then you can freeze them in grease paper. When you need them, you can defrost them, and grill until they are ready to eat.

Fish fingers can also be made the same way, and served hot. They cannot be frozen. Serve fish fingers with lemon.

The chicken nuggets that you are going to get in the market are definitely substandard. They are made up of the lowest quality meat present in battery grown chickens, and the rest of the nuggets are going to be full up with low nutrient fillers, water and salt. Do not feed your children that terrible product made up of chicken contaminated with growth enhancers.

The two recipes given above are invaluable for all those parents whose children just love hamburgers and chicken nuggets. You can fix up these items for your children, when you have time to spare, and keep them in the freezer for when you want them.

Chips

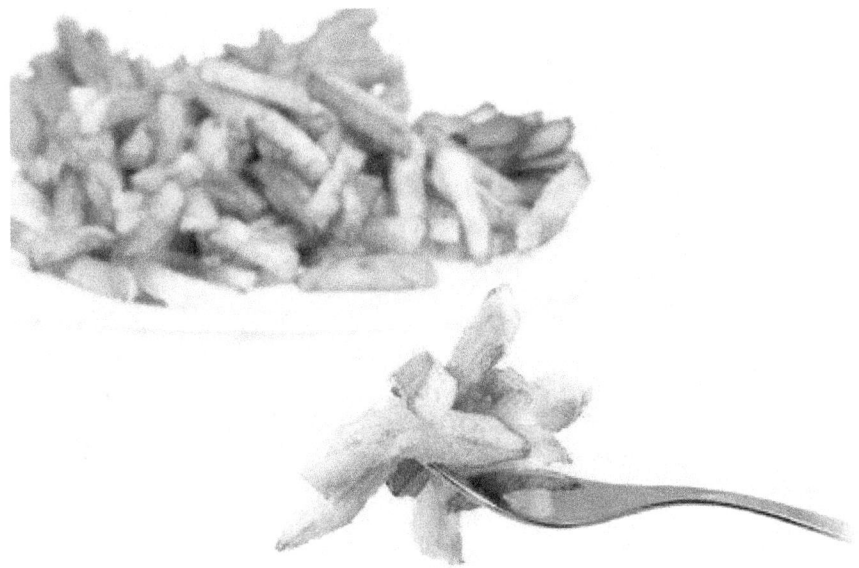

The greasy chips that you get in the market are definitely not healthy. They are also going to be inundated with salt and high sodium preservatives. Just make chips at home, – they are really easy to make – and wonder why you spend so much money buying those salty monosodium glutamate sprinkled chips.

Choose potatoes, which are normally used for baking. Scrub them clean. You do not need to remove the skin. Chop them into chips. Put a single layer on your baking tray, and brush a little olive oil on their surface. Bake in a medium-high oven until they are cooked. You may need to turn once or twice with a spatula and add a little bit of oil if needed, though I would not suggest doing that. The end result should not be greasy and should be totally dry.

Do not salt. You can eat these chips by dipping them in homemade tomato ketchup or in yogurt dips.

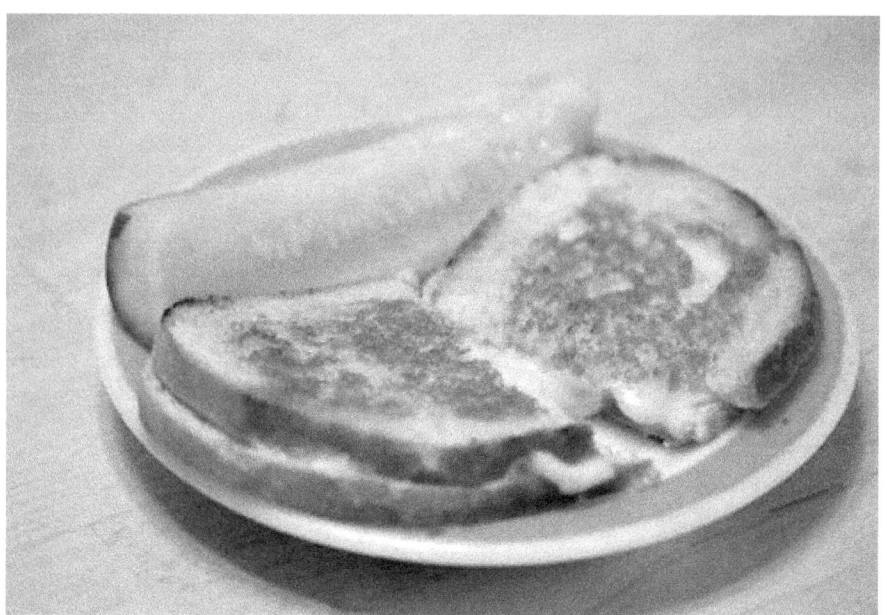

I used to enjoy grilled sandwiches very much as a kid. I still do. At that time we did not have toasters which sealed the edges of the sandwiches. Instead, we had handheld sandwich makers. This is what they looked like.

http://www.ebay.com/itm/Original-Vintage-Toas-Tite-Campfire-Sandwich-Toast-Pie-Maker-Camping-Cooker-/161437500387?pt=LH_DefaultDomain_0&hash=item25966cc3e3

I definitely do not use my vintage toaster on a campfire, but on my kitchen stove. I just take two pieces of bread, and make the filling of boiled eggs, tomato, onion, chopped and cooked minced meat, chicken, cooked vegetables, and anything else which I can imagine.

Then I place it on the fire, allow the toast to cook for less than a minute, turn over, let the other side cook, and there I am, a hot grilled sandwich ready to eat with ketchup, tomatoes, spring onions, red pepper, or anything else which is in the fridge.

Ice cream

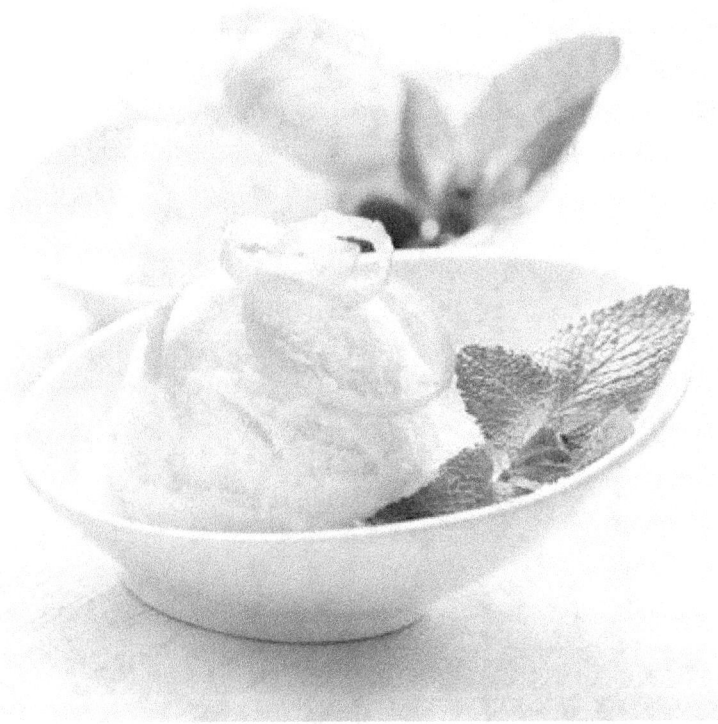

What is the fun of enjoying your childhood, if you cannot have plenty of ice cream. A scoop or two of ice cream is always welcome, as long as it is not smothered in gooey sauces and toppings, which are rich in sugar and artificial coloring.

Conclusion

Childhood obesity is getting to be a worldwide problem, especially in developed and developing countries, where lifestyle changes are affecting the general health of children. So healthy dietary habits have to be the priority of responsible parents to make sure that children are fed healthy meals, and do not suffer from obesity.

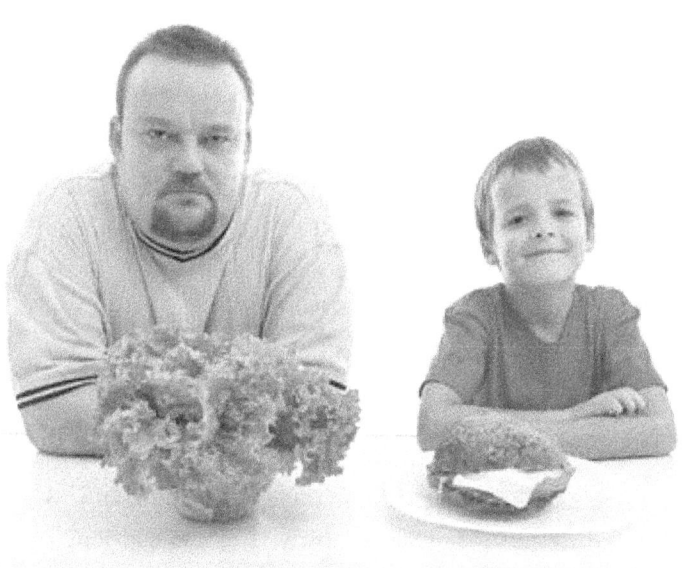

Remember that the health of your family is your responsibility. So here is one good idea in order to make your child more adventurous in eating. Avoid putting him off with your own prejudices, dislikes and expectations. Ask him to taste a new dish at least once, because it is possible that he is going to find it tasty, even if you found it horrible and yucky.

You will need to lead by example here. Healthy eating can be encouraged by eating fresh food. Food which is perishable, and has not been properly refrigerated may cause food poisoning. So once a child falls sick after eating one particular food item, he is never going to touch it again. So use some common sense, give your children fresh fruit and freshly cooked food.

Look at foodstuffs which have high nutritional value. Children suffering from overweight and obesity problems have, in most cases their parents to blame for their bad health. That is because the parents enjoy eating, especially without bothering about the nutritive value of the food being eaten in such large amounts.

The children follow suit, thinking it normal to eat food in large quantities, just like their parents do. What they do not realize is that their parents are fully grown adults, with a strong digestive system. A growing child still needs to reach the stage when his system can managed to assimilate food in large quantities.

So if you overfeed your baby, he is going to turn out obese. And then when he sees you eating lots of food, as he grows out of babydom, and into childhood, he is going to think it normal to eat whatever comes at hand and at odd times.

Children are going to learn by observation and they are likely to eat a wide variety of foods if they see their parents doing so on a regular basis. Do not enforce eating habits, especially with streams of instructions being shouted out at the children like *eat your vegetables, they are good for you, keep your elbows off the table, use your fork and knife, not your fingers* and so on.

Instead, create a pleasant and relaxed atmosphere, while you are eating with your children and teaches them behavior codes which they are going to learn through observation.

If you are unable to sit down together with your children for meals on a daily basis, being very busy, make it a point of doing so, at least once or twice at weekends. During the week, just sit down with your children when they are eating and eat or drink something whenever you are able to. This is to make sure that they are not left alone when they are eating, or they are relegated to eating with other children. Consider it quality time.

You may not think this to be a major part of bringing up children, but your children are some consciously going to feel more secure, especially when you spend most of your time working.

My sister-in-law is a working lady. But she makes it a point to be at home, when her children come home from school in the afternoon. The moment they come in, hungry as little bears at lunchtime, there she is, sitting on the table, ready to dish up lunch, and asking them about how their day went.

 I asked her how she managed that, and she said, "I always take up jobs where I can get home when they come home from school. I tell my boss that if he wants me in the evenings, I would be willing to work as long as the lunchtime, which I consider to be a sacred time with my children is free."

How many mothers have the time or the inclination to do that? Once upon time, in the 20th century, mothers used to do just that. But nowadays, the 21st century has latch key kids, coming home to an empty house. This is a sad state of affairs, which is getting to be more and more prevalent all over the world. The idea of "quality time" to interact with your own children is frankly speaking terrible.

Child rearing, an important parental responsibility cannot be slotted into 15 minute intervals of "hello, my child, how are you, how was your day", before rushing off to your next appointment. And when your child wants to talk to you, you say "I am too busy, ask your father/mother." And forget about him.

In such cases, do not blame others for your children to grow up emotionally deprived, and could not caring less about you, when he grows up.

So your priority is to keep yourself healthy. It is also to make sure that your child is healthy and happy.

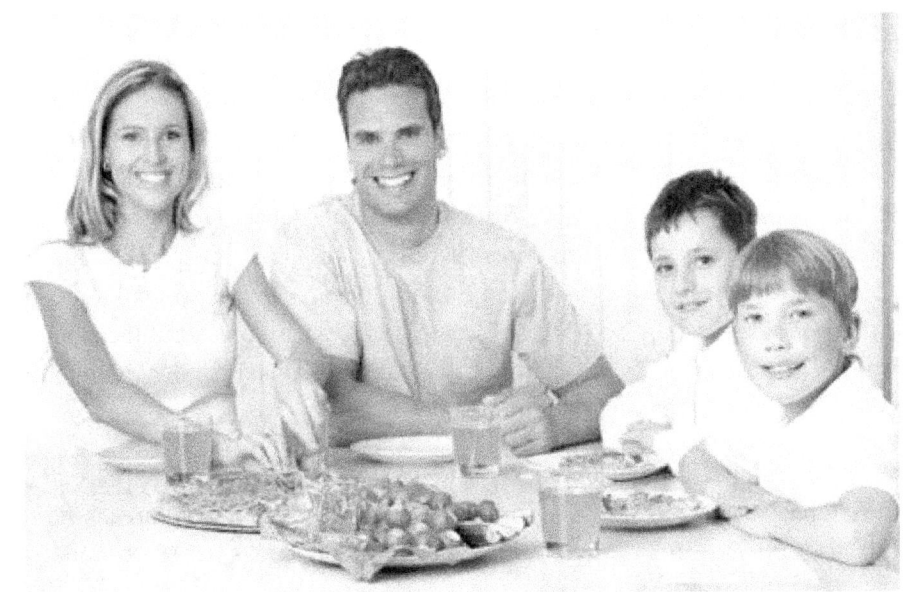

I hope that was orange juice and not an orange flavored soft drink…

Live Long and Prosper!

Authors Bio-

Dueep Jyot Singh is a Management and IT Professional who managed to gather Postgraduate qualifications in Management and English and Degrees in Science, French and Education while pursuing different enjoyable career options like being an hospital administrator, IT,SEO and HRD Database Manager/ trainer, movie , radio and TV scriptwriter, theatre artiste and public speaker, lecturer in French, Marketing and Advertising, ex-Editor of Hearts On Fire (now known as Solstice) Books Missouri USA, advice columnist and cartoonist, publisher and Aviation School trainer, ex- moderator on Medico.in, banker, student councilor ,travelogue writer ... among other things!

One fine morning, she decided that she had enough of killing herself by Degrees and went back to her first love -- writing. It's more enjoyable! She already has 48 published academic and 14 fiction- in- different- genre books under her belt.

When she is not designing websites or making Graphic design illustrations for clients , she is browsing through old bookshops hunting for treasures, of which she has an enviable collection – including R.L. Stevenson, O.Henry, Dornford Yates, Maurice Walsh, De Maupassant, Victor Hugo, Sapper, C.N. Williamson, "Bartimeus" and the crown of her collection- Dickens "The Old Curiosity Shop," and so on... Just call her "Renaissance Woman") - collecting herbal remedies, acting like Universal Helping Hand/Agony Aunt, or escaping to her dear mountains for a bit of exploring, collecting herbs and plants and trekking.

Our books are available at

1. Amazon.com
2. Barnes and Noble
3. Itunes
4. Kobo
5. Smashwords
6. Google Play Books

Check out some of the other JD-Biz Publishing books
Gardening Series on Amazon

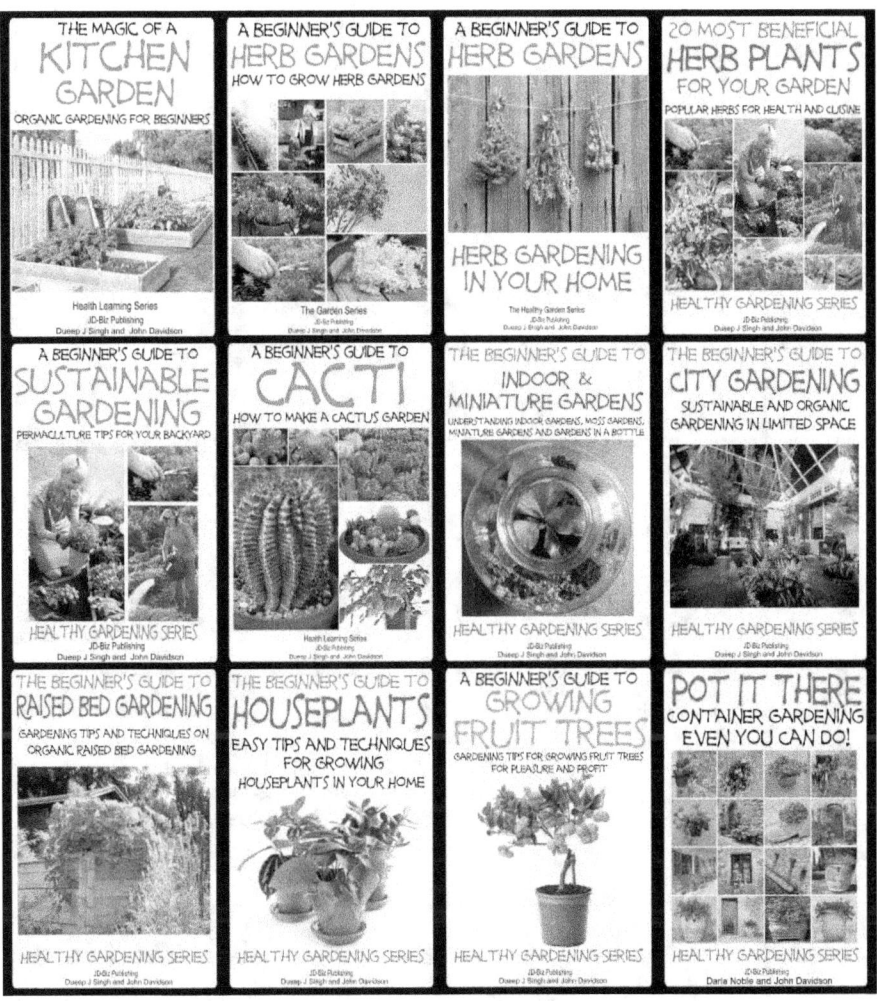

Health Learning Series

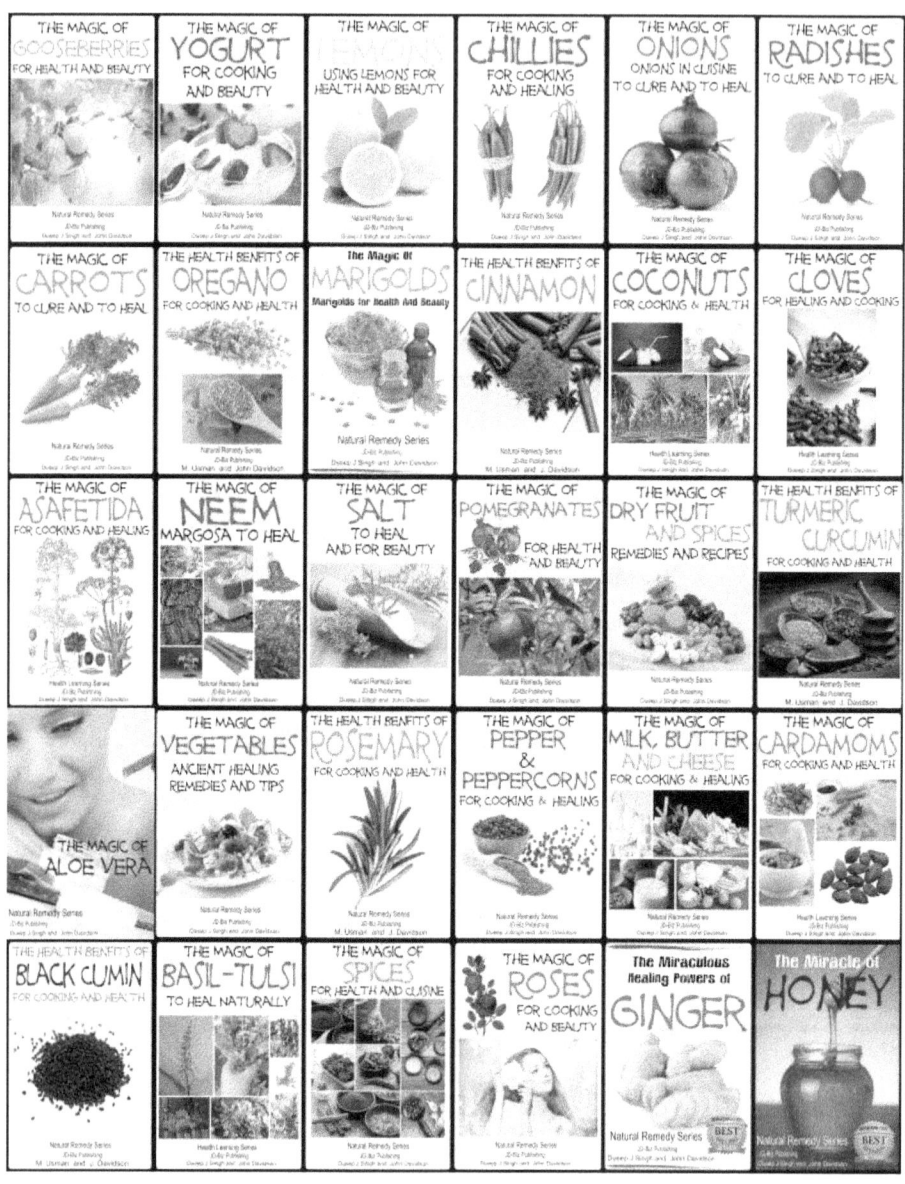

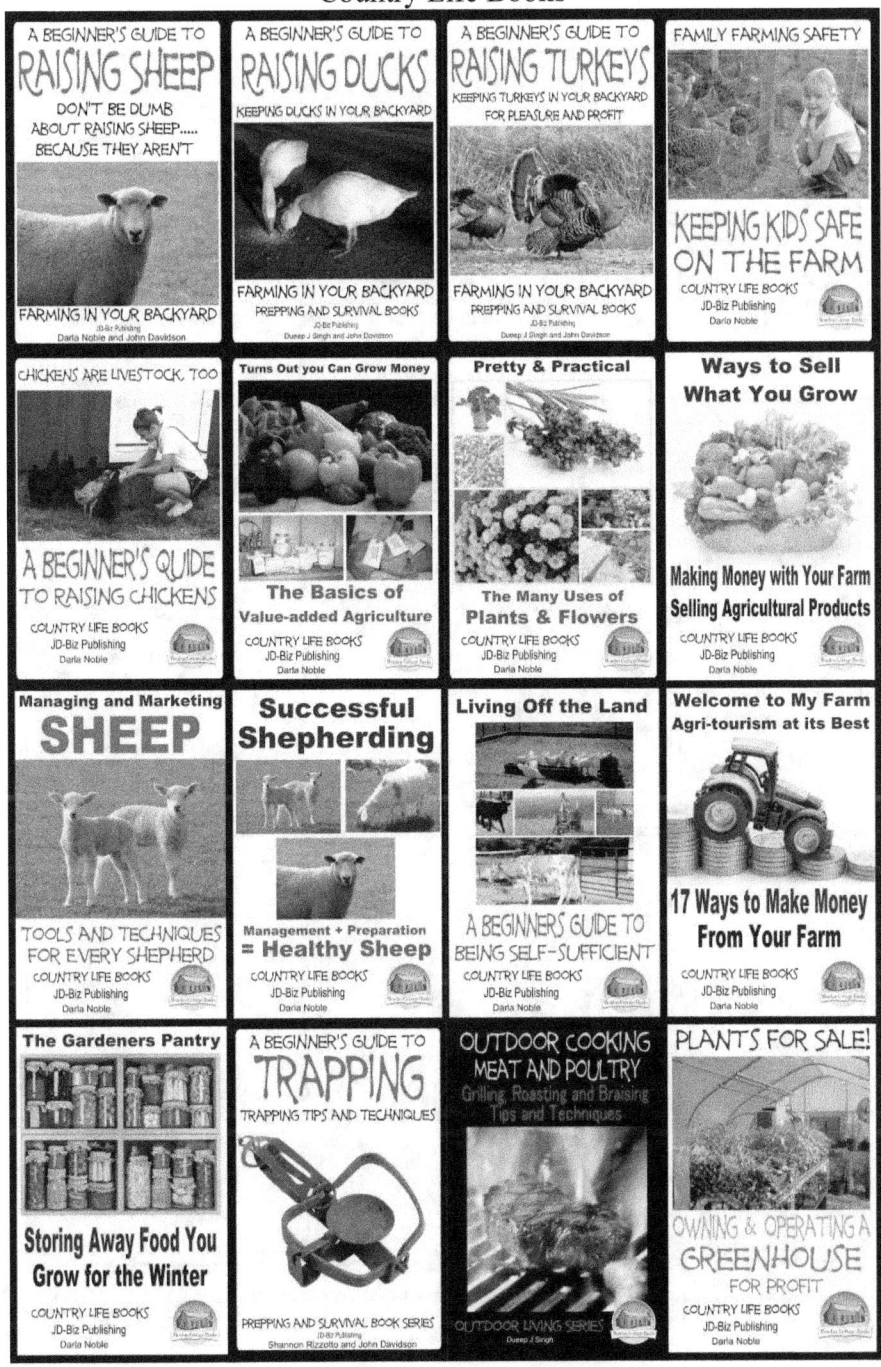

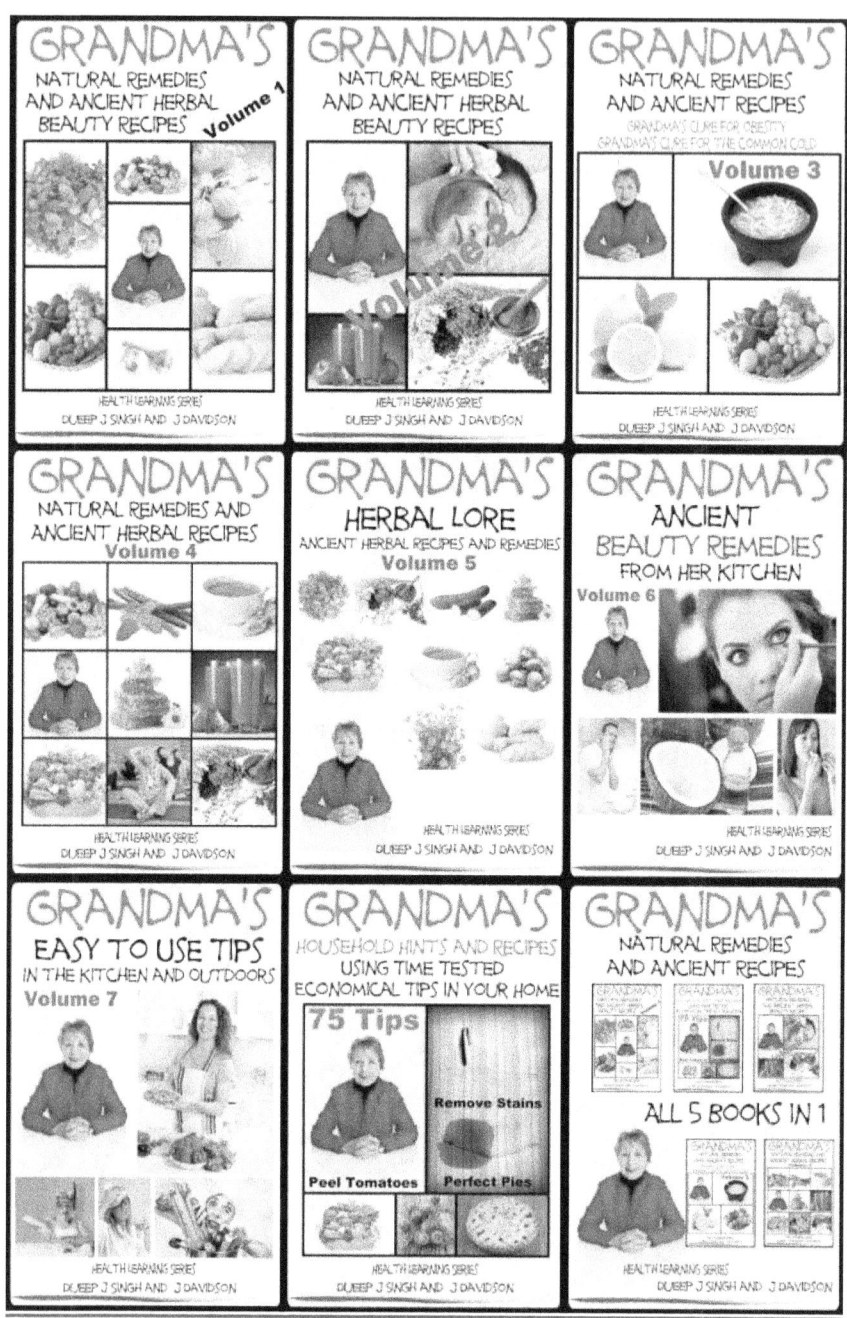

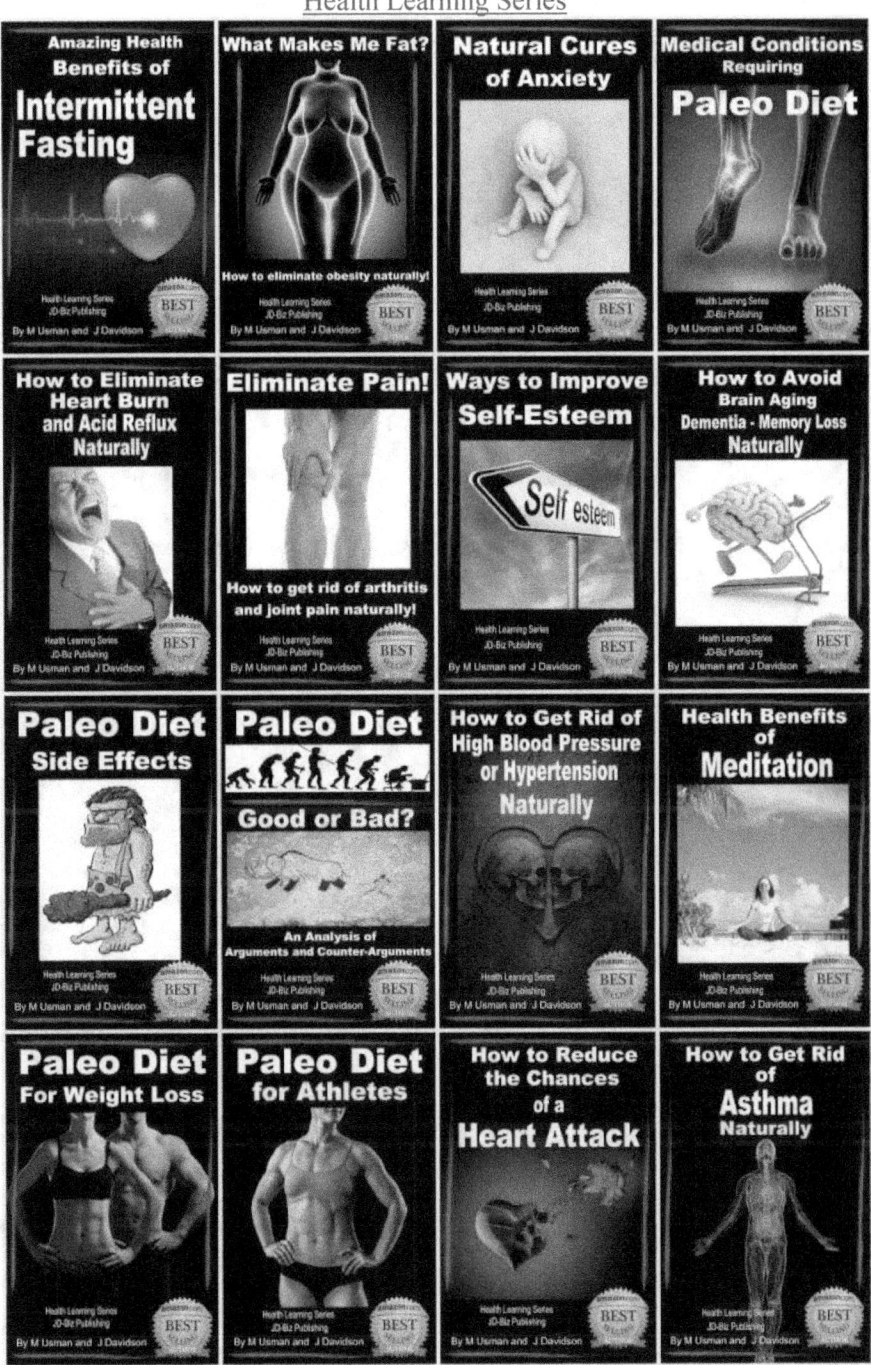

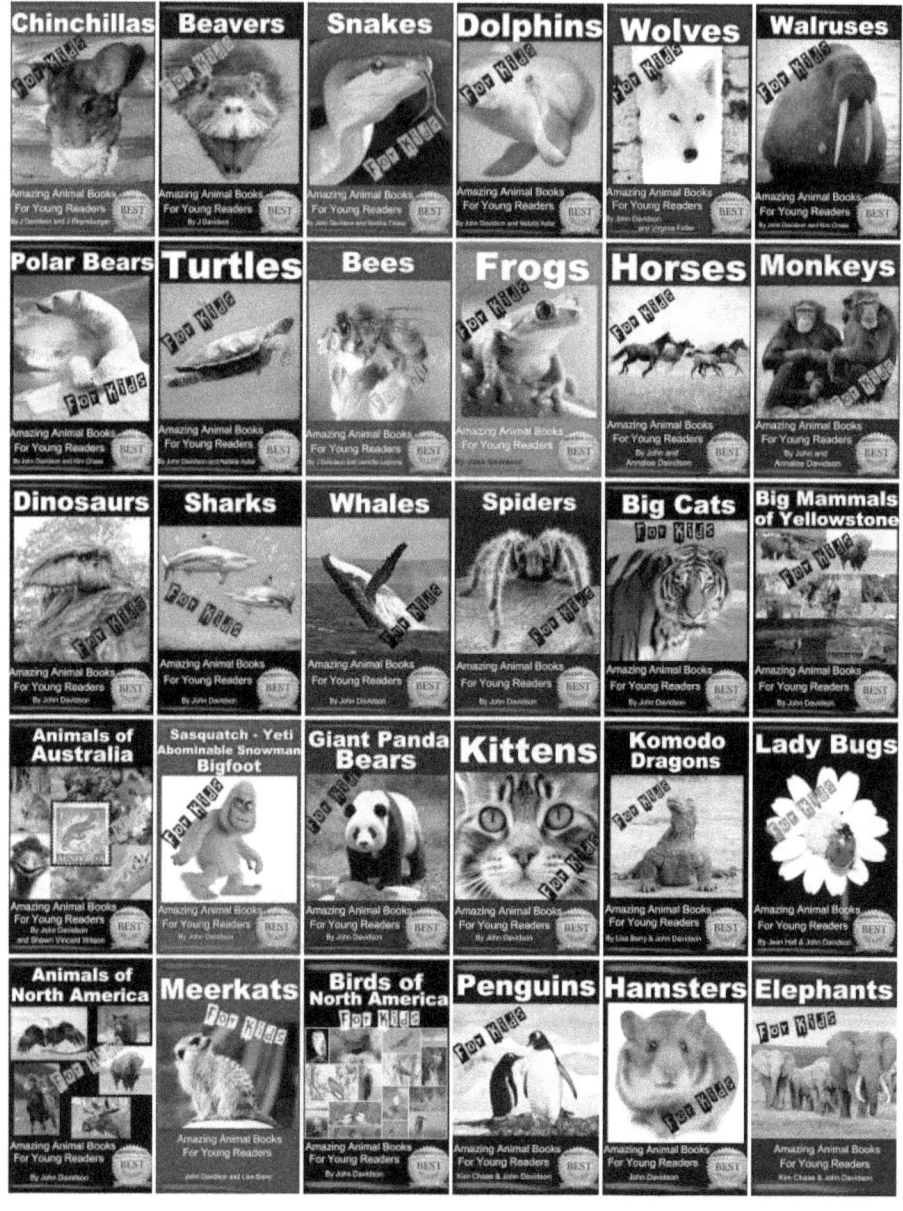

Learn To Draw Series

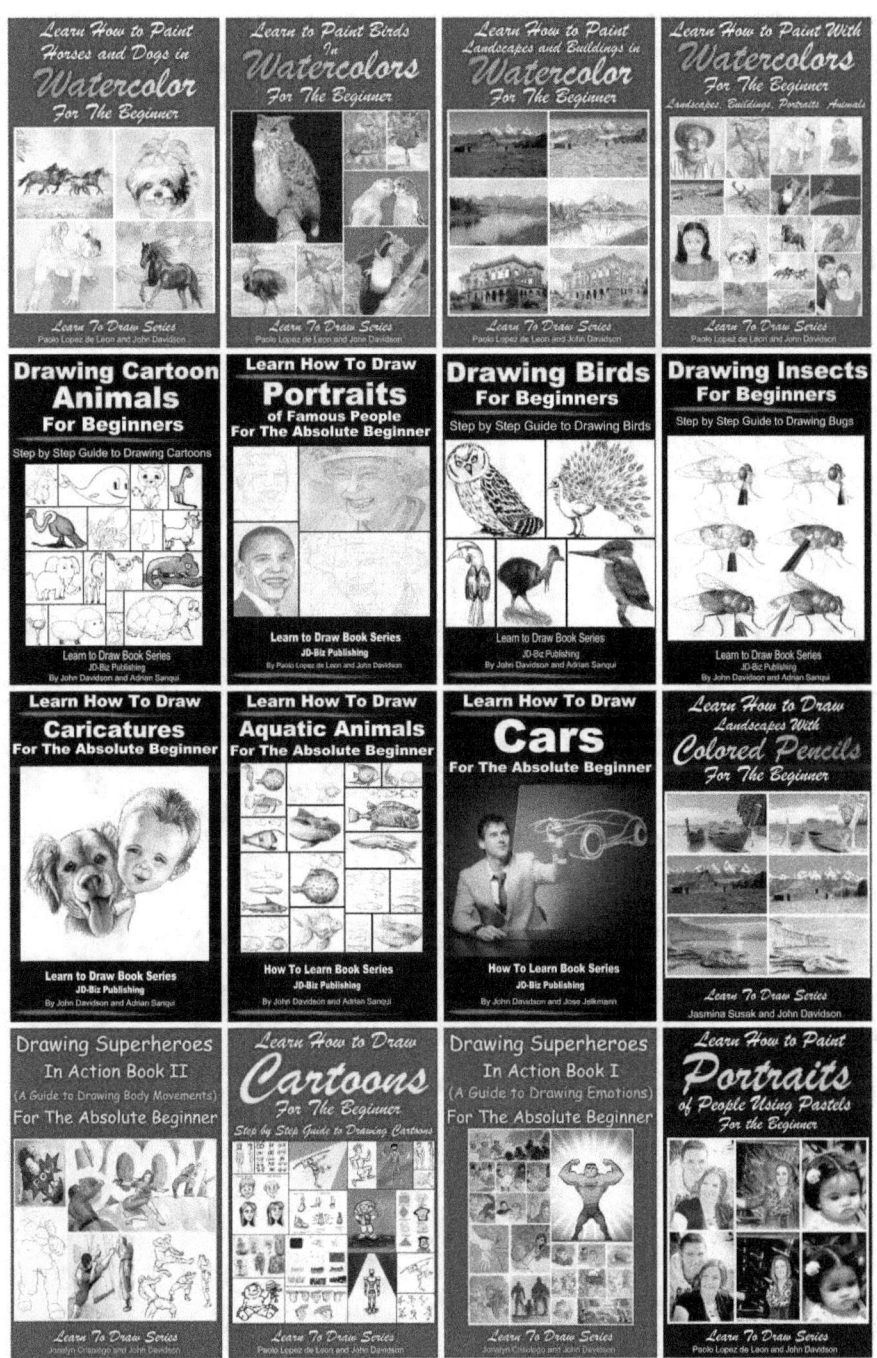

How to Build and Plan Books

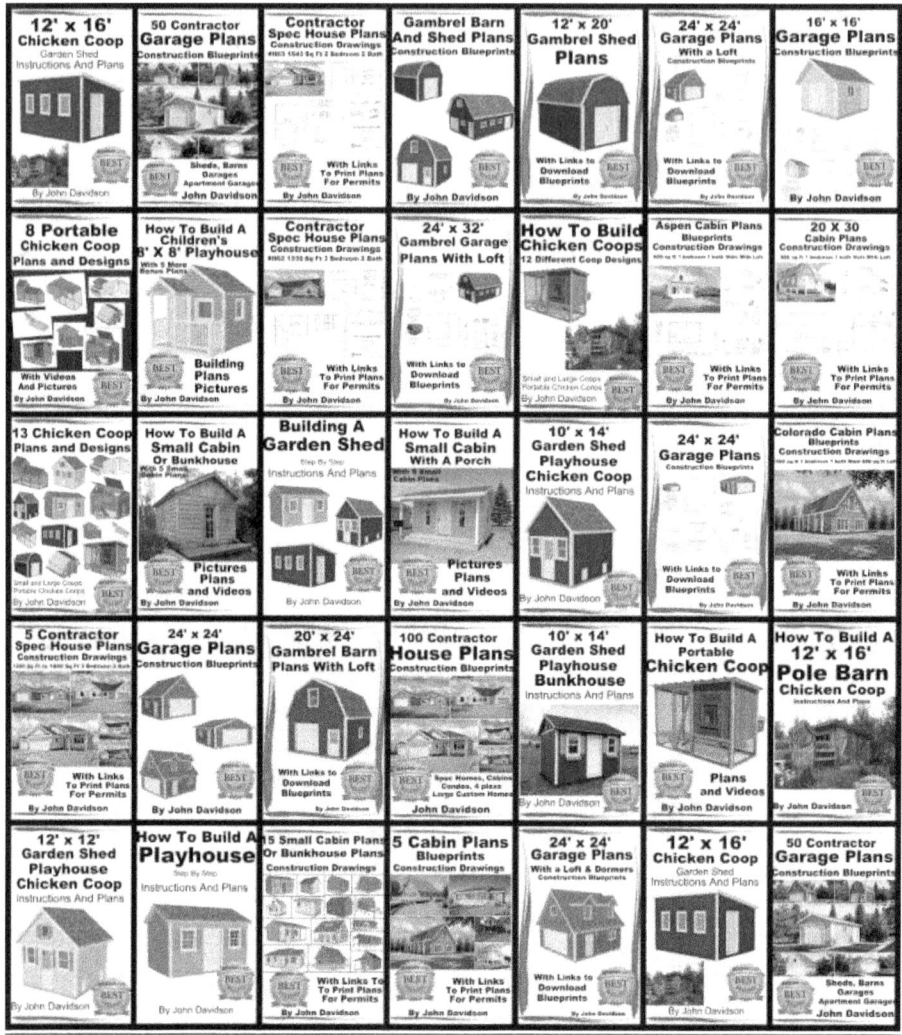

Entrepreneur Book Series

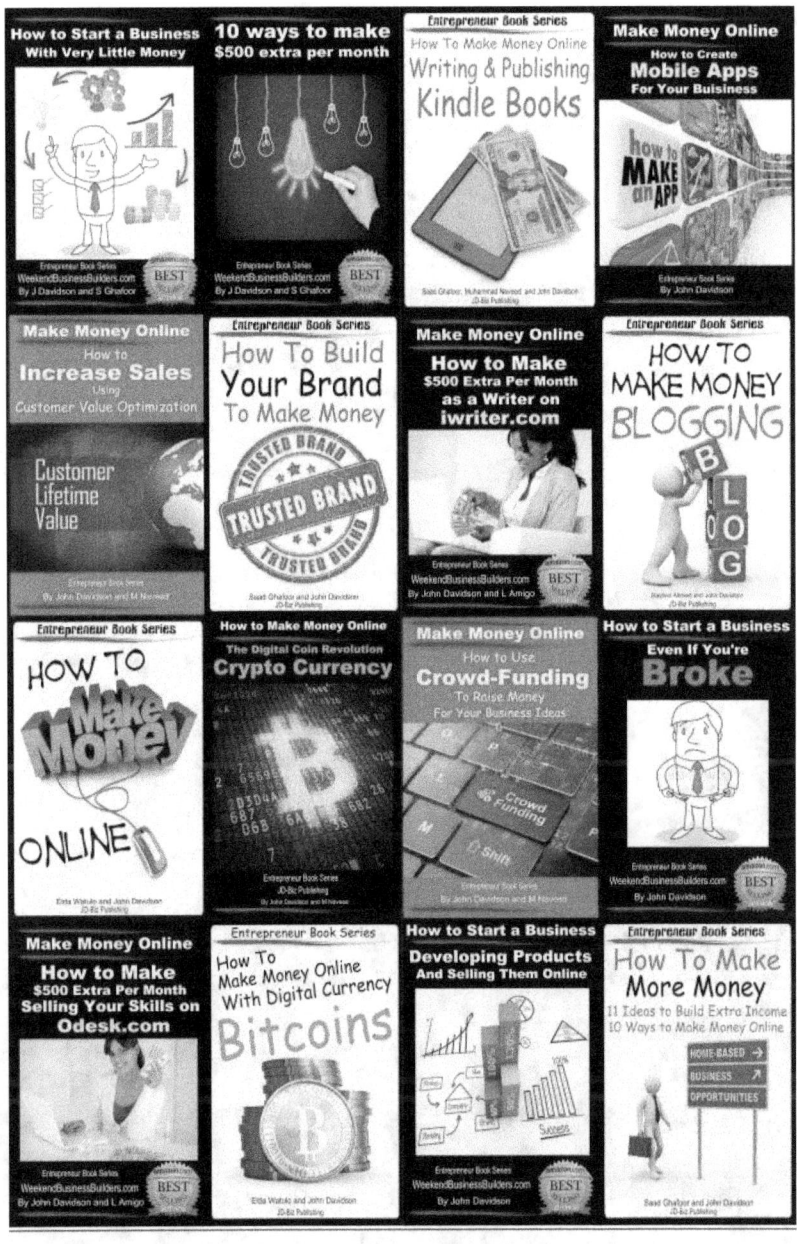

Publisher

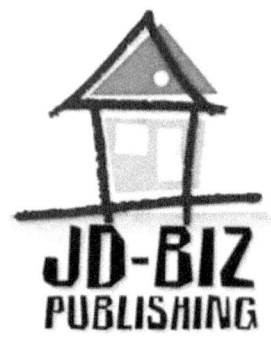

JD-Biz Corp

P O Box 374

Mendon, Utah 84325

http://www.jd-biz.com/

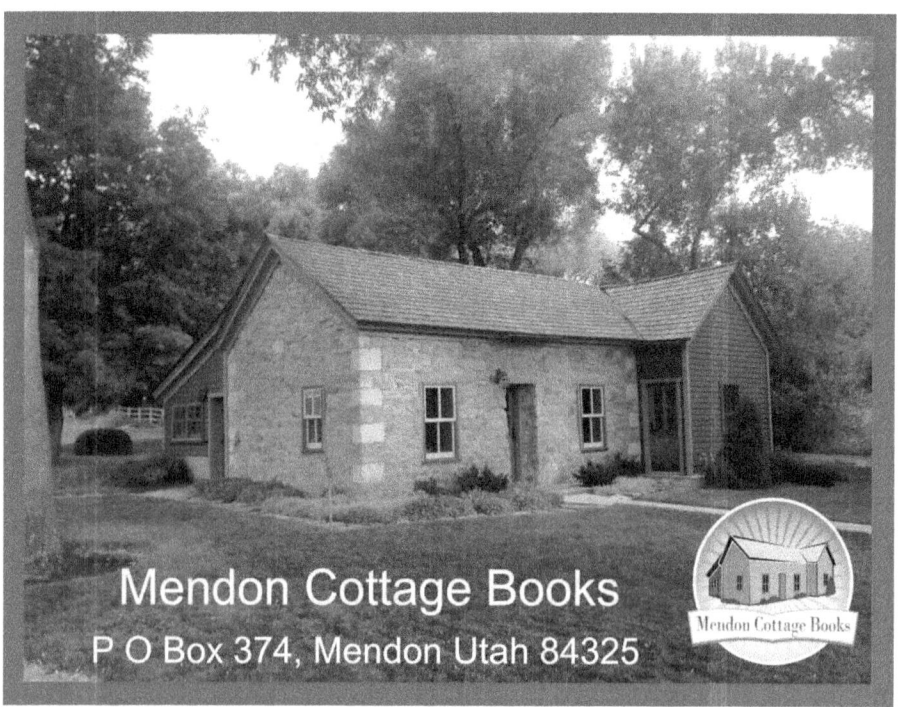

Mendon Cottage Books
P O Box 374, Mendon Utah 84325

www.ingramcontent.com/pod-product-compliance
Lightning Source LLC
Chambersburg PA
CBHW071144280526
45787CB00003B/1403